New Healing Secrets of Angels and Herbs

by Jennifer Bailey

BALBOA.
PRESS

A DIVISION OF HAY HOUSE

Balboa Press books may be ordered through booksellers or by contacting:

Balboa Press
A Division of Hay House
1663 Liberty Drive
Bloomington, IN 47403
www.balboapress.com.au
1-(877) 407-4847

ISBN: 978-1-4525-0928-0 (sc)
ISBN: 978-1-4525-0929-7 (e)

Because of the dynamic nature of the Internet, any web addresses or links contained in this book may have changed since publication and may no longer be valid. The views expressed in this work are solely those of the author and do not necessarily reflect the views of the publisher, and the publisher hereby disclaims any responsibility for them.

The author of this book does not dispense medical advice or prescribe the use of any technique as a form of treatment for physical, emotional, or medical problems without the advice of a physician, either directly or indirectly. The intent of the author is only to offer information of a general nature to help you in your quest for emotional and spiritual well-being. In the event you use any of the information in this book for yourself, which is your constitutional right, the author and the publisher assume no responsibility for your actions.

Any people depicted in stock imagery provided by Thinkstock are models, and such images are being used for illustrative purposes only.
Certain stock imagery © Thinkstock.

Printed in the United States of America

Balboa Press rev. date: 03/26/2013

CONTENTS

INTRODUCTION

Angels of the light, Beings of light and love, and the Fairy kingdom are now flowing closer to us, to assist everyone in every way they can. With the new doorways opening, and with the changes in the energies of the planets and the solar system, other wondrous changes are also happening.

We know that the Sun, and Moon affects all living things on Earth, but now the Angels are channeling energies from the planets, constellations, and stars, through the matrix of the growing herbs. These energies are cleansing and enlivening the crystal grids, and the biochemical pathways of the herbs, and revitalizing their life force. It is truly an exciting time. The Angels are delighted, because they want these energies to also flow to us, to cleanse and vitalize our crystal grid, to enliven our biochemical pathways, and to increase our spiritual awareness and knowledge, for 2012 and beyond.

Having always grown and used fresh herbs all my life, and as an herbalist working with patients for over 26 years, I have always felt that something more was happening than just the medicinal qualities and the mineral content of the herbs healing people. There seemed to be a spark of vitality, a vibrant energy affecting them as well. Having taught meditation as a teacher for over 20 years, I was often given information as to how the herbs were working in the body, the organs and the cells. But, I was amazed when the Angels expressed their desire to bring to Earth, new spiritual energies, to help us, in this new Aquarian age as it is unfolding. They also requested that this information be available to everyone, to use with their families, pets and gardens.

With so many chemicals and toxins in the ground, the air, the water, and our foods, help is now desperately needed. These chemicals not only contribute to major health and environmental problems, as never seen before, they can alter the structure of our cells, organs, and biochemical pathways. The toxins can also block our spiritual energies, and our crystal matrix, and hold us in our lower chakras and keep us blocked. This is stopping us being beautiful, strong, radiant life force beings, reaching our full potential and becoming who we are meant to be. Not only, can we eat healthy organic fruit, vegetables and food, to strengthen our whole being, we can now also channel spiritual energies and colours, from the assigned Angel, Fairy and plant deva associated to each herb.

During the times of Atlantis, in the healing temples, beautiful Angels used sound, crystals, medicinal herbs and colours to finely tune our chakras, bodies, mind, and spirit, so that our emotions could be balanced, blocks could be removed, and gentle healing could take place. Now, some of this information is being revealed, so that our spiritual knowledge from Atlantis can be remembered, and our 12 strand DNA can be awakened.

By starting to use these herbs, colours and crystals in our own home and garden, we are also creating one small paradise for the plant devas, sprites, and elemental kingdoms to return to the earth, to cleanse the ground, the air and the water. You never know, you may start to see them. One garden creates one Eden, one light, one powerhouse of positive energy, which can flow out into the neighbouring area. What a wonderful gift we have at our fingertips, even if we only use this knowledge ourselves to feel more energetic, more nourished, and more vitalized. I have started using the herb teas, the commands, the colours, and the angels myself, and with patients and friends, and the results have been astounding. Let's make a difference in this world! After all a huge lake can start with only one drop of water!

Having lovingly tended an herb garden for most of my life and watched with delight as all the butterflies, bees, birds and insects swarmed around the flowers and herbs, I am immensely overjoyed at this new information, and the chance to encourage all of us to grow and use the herbs, for our own health and enjoyment. But how amazing it is also for us to work with the Angels, Fairies, the plant devas and their spiritual energies.

MY JOURNEY

Wondrous stories of pixies, fairies, and sprites were a large part of our lives when I was a child. Stories of gum-nut blossom babies, flower fairies and tree spirits, all seemed so real at the time and sparked our imaginations and dreams.

Growing up on a farm, surrounded constantly by brightly coloured birds, parrots, butterflies, dragonflies, beetles, native wildlife and plants, life seemed like a beautiful mystery of the universe. There it was, all around me.

I was lucky that my father and I would wake at dawn and walk through the lanes for miles to gather the sheep. We'd watch the sun rise, with its pastel pinks and lilacs painting the sky and sending rays of colour across the land, bathing all in its pathway. The colours would slowly change hues, moving to bright oranges and golden yellows. All the while, my father would point out all the native plants, flowers, birds, and animals and their secret hiding places. It was so peaceful and delightful with the sun streaming golden rays of light through the leaves and trees. But best of all were the tall Red Gum trees with their massive girths and spotted trunks. The trees were filled with millions of thriving insects, caterpillars, singing cicadas, spiders, and birds. It was like a village unto itself.

My mother was a passionate gardener with a voracious appetite for growing flowers, trees, vegetables and exotic fruit. However it was when she took my sister and me, wandering over the paddocks collecting delicious field mushrooms, that she told us stories of the gum-nut blossom babies. Whenever we asked her how to see them, she'd say we would have to tiptoe and sneak up on the blossoms ever so quietly. But they must've always heard us, because when we got close, they had already disappeared. We'd wrap our arms around the huge trees and feel their strong radiating energies.

I kept these memories within me, and many years later I laughed at how we thought about the plants and flowers as homes for the fairies.

However, a few years ago, many miles from home, I stayed in the rainforest to do a meditation training course. One meditation was to visualize walking through the trees and being given a sign as to what we should do in our lives. My mind was suddenly out in the rainforest, and immediately a 4ft. Fairy King and Queen appeared before me. They explained that they wanted to come forward now to work with people to help the Earth, the plants and the environment. Feeling quite amazed and astounded, I wondered who that would be. A few years later they appeared to me again and said people were ready for the Fairies and the Angels to give us new information on what to do. It was this which has started my journey. I was to channel their information, write it down, and pass this knowledge on to others. Now, we can all work together to heal and cleanse the crystal grid of the earth, and to help cleanse the earth of the toxins and chemicals which have been carelessly saturating the planet, the air, the water and the environment.

Because the big picture is overwhelming, the Angels and the Fairies are showing us how to start in our own gardens. Remember, many tiny stars make up the night sky which can light up the whole planet. We can be individual stars lighting up our own back yards, paving the way for the Angels to work with us now, so that every small area is unblocking and cleansing the Earth's energy grid. The Earth's grid must be cleansed so that the ley lines, and spiritual pathways in the earth can eventually connect up, as they were during Atlantis. Then the spiritual grids between the pyramids, Uluru, Stonehenge, Glastonbury, and other sacred sites around the world, will once more be places of greater, sacred, spiritual power.

The Angels, Fairies, and plant devas would love it if we only used natural sprays, such as garlic and other herbs to repel unwanted insects. However we can also ask the Angels, Fairies and plant devas to protect them, use white light, other colours, solar radiance, companion planting or homeopathic sprays. There are endless ways. Although the information, in this book may now help the plants, the birds, the animals, ourselves, and our families, it can also be helping the earth. Let's have fun, the Angels and Fairies are ready to work with you now!

INTRODUCTION TO THE HERBS

The Herbs have been grouped into families, and this helps, because family groups have similar properties. For example the Labiatae family like sage and thyme are antiseptic, so are good for colds and 'flu. One time, when my mother had a shocking cold but the farm's garden only had oregano and marjoram growing, (both in the Labiatae plant family) I made her a tea with the herbs and honey. She was so surprised how the tea helped her cold so quickly.

Although there are many herbs, the Beings of Light have requested that I write about the most popular ones, as we can easily grow them and use them without being overwhelmed by too many.

Initially it is very important to do the meditation with each herb, colour, Angel, Fairy and plant deva, to introduce yourself to them, associate with them, and sense how you feel. I love these exercises, and the more we practise them, and bring the Angels in, the quicker the body and cells will respond to them, and then healing can take place. If you are very sick in bed you may spend hours doing the meditations, and talking to the Angels and Fairies. However when you are in a hurry, drinking an herb tea at home or at work, the affirmation at the bottom of each herb page, can be said quickly to reinforce the healing energies. Several herbs may be used together in a teapot, or cup, such as Sage and Thyme for colds, sore throat and coughs. Rosemary and Sage combined are good for memory, studying, energy, and focus, and Calendula and Yarrow, for wound healing, ulcers, or soothing cystitis. Try them!

On the first page for each herb, the top section shows the official Latin name, the part of the plant which is used, the medicinal actions, and the medicinal indications. These can be found in any herb text book, (probably since Greek and Roman times) and were also explained to me at college by my teachers. The lower section of the page shows the Angels and Fairies now associated with each herb, and the new energies and qualities they are bringing in with that specific herb. So please enjoy growing and using your herbs, practise the meditations with the Angels, Fairies, and colours, and feel the energy, vitality and the difference in your health!

ANGELS & FAIRIES HEALING WITH THE HERBS

HERB	MEANING	ARCHANGEL	FAIRY	COLOUR
Boraginacea				
Borage	Congestion	Uriel	Queen Titiana	Lilac, cream, violet
Comfrey	Scar healing	Raphiel	Queen Gwynneth	Blue/green
Compositaea				
Calendula	Purifier	Surion	Queen Stellari	White, golden yellow
Chamomile	Soothing	Chamuel	Queen Aerielle	Light blue, light indigo
Chicory	Accepting	Samuel	Queen Chisarka	Light blue, pale lemon
Dandelion	Detoxer	Metatron	King Letophile	Gold with gold and silver sparkles
Labiatae				
Lavender	Self Heal	Gabriel	Queen Lelitha	Violet
Lemon Balm	Calming	Oriel	Queen Aurora	White, pale blue
Peppermint	Stimulating	Sophiel	Queen Philipa	Light lime green
Rosemary	Energising	Zadkiel	Queen Marella	Bright orange
Sage	Knowing	Chakriel	King Wultter	Dark red, Light blue
Thyme	Expeller	Fadkiel	King Tanuk & Queen Aurora	Light yellow, violet
Liliacea				
Garlic	Antiseptic	Anturian	King Solaris	Bright golden yellow
Rosacea				
Raspberry	Blood tonic	Uriel	Queen Anaphiel	Ruby red
Umbelliferae				
Dill	Contentment	Suriel	King Favriel	Silvery light blue
Fennel	Dispeller	Zaniel	Queen Floriad	Citrus greenyellow
Parsley	Releaser	Savarone	Queen Faverell	Bright yellow green
Yarrow	Wound healer	Michael	King Santonelle & Queen florissa	White, light pink

BORAGINACEA HERBS

BORAGE —(Borago officinalis)

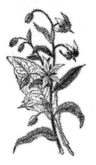

Part used: root, leaf, flowers.

Flower: purple star-shaped flower.

Actions: Diaphoretic, galactogogue, expectorant.

Indications: Borage has similar properties to Comfrey. It aids in fevers, and pleurisy, and strengthens the lungs. A tea with the leaves helps the flow of lactating mother's milk. Borage is a restorative agent to the adrenal glands.

ANGEL: **Archangel Uriel.**

FAIRY: **Queen Titiana.**

WORD: **Congestion.**

Uses: Although Comfrey works more on the crystalline and ethereal level, Borage goes deeper in to remove hardened or stubborn congestion, mucous, phlegm, pus, and rubbish in the body, especially the lungs. As the lungs are one of the first contacts the internal body has with the outside air, gases and contaminants, the rubbish must be removed and cleared for oxygen, pure air and spiritual energies to come in. Like Comfrey, Borage helps repair networks, vessels and structure, especially the lungs. It can now help heal deep seated weaknesses in the lungs, including held in grief, trauma from wars, or horror and shock. It is nurturing on a slightly emotional level where the emotions are blocked within the cells, from childhood and from past lives. The purple flower helps with healing on a physical and spiritual level.

COLOUR: Borage energies vibrate pale lilac, cream and dark violet swirls

BORAGE

Borage is high in silica and calcium which have an affinity for breaking down mucous, as well as strengthening other tissues and cells.

It was one of the herbs the Centurians used, for its planetary energies, as well as its physical health aspects.

Although more gentle than Comfrey, it is nurturing when one is convalescing. The lungs and adrenals, often both store within them, the feelings of stress, grief and exhaustion, as well as being organs of elimination to filter out toxins. Borage supports both organs. Archangel Uriel and Fairy Queen Titiana with their love and understanding for humanity, are working together with this herb, magically weaving their spiritual energies into the matrix of Borage to help us on many levels, to strengthen our physical and spiritual bodies. They are delighted that, with the dissolving of the veils, and with the new dimensional energies of the solar system coming in, they are able to come closer to us, to love and support us. With colds and 'flu, lung problems, giving up smoking, for cellular health, and when healing is needed, place a request whilst using Borage.

"Archangel Uriel, Fairy Queen Titiana, and the plant devas of Borage, please allow your healing energies through Borage flow into my body, especially my lungs, to break down and eliminate mucous and toxins and to heal the physical structure and crystalline structure of my body and cells."

Imagine pale lilac, pale cream, and dark violet swirls flowing within your body for a few minutes whilst placing this request, and when finished, command that the colours are ceasing to flow. Then place a sincere thank-you to Archangel Uriel, Queen Titiana, and plant devas of Borage.

When placing the Borage plant in the garden or in a pot, request:

"Archangel Uriel, Fairy Queen Titiana and the plant devas pertaining to Borage please bring in the spiritual energies of the stars, and solar system which are needed now to heal, soothe, and comfort the ground, the earths crystal grid, the water, the air, the animals, birds, insects and plants, so that the healing process may start. Thank-you."

Think of a white sparkling energy flowing into the garden. A white quartz crystal or violet crystal may be placed next to Borage to help the healing processes.

Affirmation: "My lungs, adrenals and crystal grid are being strengthened and cleansed and healed."

BORAGINACEA HERBS

COMFREY — (Symphytum officinale)

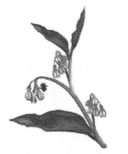

Part used: Root, leaf.

Flower: Purple tubular flowers.

Actions: vulnerary, expectorant

Indications: Comfrey contains allantoin which helps new cell growth and repair, so it aids wound healing inside the body and on the skin. Because it contains a demulcent (soothing) mucilage, it aids healing of gastric and duodenal ulcers, leg ulcers, hiatus hernias, ulcerative colitis and bladder ulcers. It strengthens the lungs, and aids expectoration of mucous, so is helpful in coughs and bronchitis. Because it is high in calcium and silica, and due to its healing properties, it is used as a poultice to help repair bone fractures.

ANGEL: **Archangel Raphael**

FAIRY: **Queen Gwynneth**

WORD: **Repair & healing**

Uses: Comfrey can heal the structure of the physical body. It also heals the crystalline structures of the bodies on all levels due to its high silica content. (ie. silica has a crystal structure) This is important for the new Crystal Children now being born. It is also needed for the crystalline structure of the earth and the planet, and to link up and energize the crystal pathways and grid. This healing herb, with its angels, will help heal bones, blood cells, the heart structure, skin, hair, the intestinal wall, the bladder structure, and veins and arteries. It will strengthen the whole body to help repel illness and microbes. Used with other herbs, it will also strengthen the aura.

COLOUR: Comfreys energies vibrate as a blue/green colour in swirls, from aqua green to the deepest green. The purple flower has the spiritual energy of the violet to strengthen the spiritual mind.

COMFREY

Comfrey was an herb used by the Celtics in olden days, due to its association with the Fairies, and its energies from Jupiter and Pluto. Comfrey was used in a lot of Celtic healing ceremonies to knit old wounds and scars, caused from old conflicts, and wars. It was also used to delve deep in, to remove old blocks and spells on the crystalline structure, so cells, tissue, bones and old wounds can repair and knit. The Chi energies and life force energies can then flow without a blockage. The fairies associated with comfrey love this herb and its flowers. They use it for themselves as well as for healing animals, birds, insects, butterflies, and plants. That is why it is good to dig the Comfrey herb into the ground where there is a dank spot or where other plants won't grow. Leave Comfrey in the ground for a few weeks to heal the area and to cleanse the earth and the water, before growing other herbs or plants there. When using this herb, even as a poultice place the request:

"May the spiritual healing energies of Archangel Raphael, Fairy Queen Gwynneth and the plant devas of Comfrey, flow within me to heal and strengthen my whole body, my bones, and all my cells and organs."

Whilst placing this request, imagine your whole body, and the area needing help, being filled with aqua blue and mid green swirls. Allow the healing to take a few minutes (although it can be longer) until you feel the difference, then place a thankyou to Archangel Raphael, Fairy Queen Gwynneth and the plant devas. Command that the colour will cease its flow.

When placing Comfrey in the garden, in a pot or the ground request:

"May Archangel Raphael, Fairy Queen Gwynneth, and the plant devas of Comfrey please awaken the earth spirits, and bring in your healing energies, so the ground may begin healing and cleansing along its crystal grid, pathways and channels. Please remove toxic chemicals, and cleanse the water, ground, air, and the surrounding garden, thankyou."

Think of aqua blue and mid green enveloping the area. You can place an aqua blue or clear quartz crystal next to Comfrey to help strengthen it, and increase the healing processes. The crystals will also strengthen the vitality of any birds, animals, earthworms, insects, and plants in your garden. This is a wonderful gift available to us.

Affirmation: "My crystal grid, whole being, and my bones are being healed, repaired and strengthened."

COMPOSITAE HERBS

CALENDULA–(Calendula officinalis)

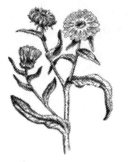

Part Used: Flower

Flower: Yellow daisy

Actions: Anti-inflammatory, anti-funghal, vulnerary, cholagogue, digestive.

Indications: Calendula is soothing to eczema, psoriasis, varicose ulcers, sunburn, bruises, strains, minor burns, scalds, cradle cap and nappy rash. It is used internally for digestive inflammations, stomach, and abdominal ulcers. It aids digestion, and is anti-funghal, internally and externally. Good for repairing for any slow healing wounds.

ANGEL: **Archangel Surion**

FAIRY: **Fairy Queen Stellari**

WORD: **Purifier**

Uses: Calendula channels the rays of the sun through it, so it purifies the body, healing deep wounds, ulcers, and putrid conditions, by the energizing and uplifting energies of the golden yellow. It vitalizes the cells to renew, regrow and regenerate them, and to heal in a stronger, more vibrant way. Calendula lets the light of the sun and the solar system lift the energy vibration of the cells and the soul, so the body can heal itself. Calendula cleans out toxins from the digestive tract and liver so they can both work more efficiently. It can also help clear out stagnant hurt or jealous emotions from the liver. It heals old scars and ulcers. Calendula can also strengthen the eyes to remove cloudiness, to be able to see things more clearly on a higher level. Calendula will also bring the fairies into the garden and the earth for healing, and to remove toxins, dangerous microbes and stagnant energies. Thus the soil is then renewed and re-energized for all the fairies, and the earth, fire, water and air devas to be able to come in and tend all the plants.

COLOUR: Calendula vibrates with bright white and golden yellow swirls.

CALENDULA

Calendula, by channeling the yellow energies of the sun through it, purifies as well as revitalizes the cells. It is especially helpful at this time for light-workers, helpers, healers, mothers, parents, and carers, who are feeling tired, exhausted and run down. With the changing energies taking place, our own bodies need strengthening, nurturing and supporting, so we can use plenty of fresh calendula flowers in salads and herbal teas, and request;

"Archangel Surion, Fairy Queen Stellari, plant devas of Calendula please allow your healing energies through Calendula flow and increase within me to purify, strengthen, and repair my body, cells and spirit."

Whilst placing this request, imagine a sunny yellow colour flowing into your whole body and aura to purify and strengthen your whole being. When you feel strengthened and balanced, command the yellow colour to cease flowing and place a thank-you to Archangel Surion, Fairy Queen Stellari and the plant devas.

Bring calendula flowers into the house, and place in a bowl or vase of water to purify the air. When planting Calendula in the garden or pot, request:

"Archangel Surion, Fairy Queen Stellari, and plant deva of Calendula please allow the spiritual energies of the sun and Calendula flow into the garden to purify, cleanse, and heal the ground, air, water, birds, animals, insects and other plants. May the devas of the garden be awakened and nourished to begin the healing processes needed by Earth at this time." Then place a sincere thank-you.

A yellow crystal or white quartz crystal may be placed next to the Calendula plant to help strengthen the healing processes taking place.

Affirmation: "The energies of Calendula and the sun are flowing into me to heal, strengthen, and vitalize my whole being."

COMPOSITAE HERBS

CHAMOMILE—(Anthemis nobile, Matricaria chamomilla)

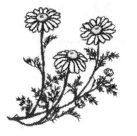

Part Used: Flower

Flower: small white daisy, with yellow centre

Actions: Antispasmodic, carminative, analgesic, antiseptic, anti-inflammatory

Indications: Chamomile is high in magnesium, so calms the stomach and reduces cramps and spasms. By relaxing and calming it aids insomnia and anxiety. It is soothing to the digestive tract so helpful in inflammation, gastritis, nausea, morning and travel sickness, dyspepsia and colic. It reduces inflammation in gingivitis and used as an eyewash to soothe sore tired eyes and conjunctivitis. Externally, it can aid with Calendula and Yarrow to soothe sunburn, psoriasis, and aid wound healing. For lactating mothers using the tea, Chamomile will help to soothe the babies to ease colic and upset tummies.

ANGEL: **Archangel Chamuel**

FAIRY: **Queen Aerielle**

WORD: **Soothing**

Uses: Chamomile, being high in magnesium, soothes children's nerves, emotions, tummies and bodies. By bringing the bodies into alignment, so there is no discourse, and by allowing the higher mind to come into the physical mind, it enables children, animals and adults to think more clearly and evenly. Bringing the bodies into alignment allows the energies to flow between them properly, and also helps to dispel anger, and irritability aggravated by the unbalanced bodies. Chamomile contains energies of Jupiter and Venus and of a distant stellar constellation to soothe and calm our bodies. It can soothe and calm deep seated angry or grey emotions held in the earth. After drinking Chamomile, use Calendula to create gentle healing and upliftment. Chamomile soothes acid, nausea, spasms and cramps, and soothes nerve signals feeding into the spine.

COLOUR: Chamomile vibrates with a light blue and light indigo swirl.

CHAMOMILE

Chamomile is one of the major herbs needed now, to grow in the garden, to soothe the static emotions building up at this time. With the upheaval of the earth's own energies, wanting to cleanse and expel any unwanted energies, planet earth also needs soothing and nurturing.

Chamomile is able to bring some of the positive energies of Jupiter and Venus into the garden for balance. Beings from these planets are now coming forward to help as much as possible, so when drinking chamomile tea or putting the flowers in a salad, or even sitting next to the plant, please request:

"Archangel Chamuel, Fairy Queen Aerielle, and the plant deva of Chamomile, please allow your spiritual energies, and the positive energies of Jupiter, and Venus contained within them, to flow into my body to soothe, and calm my body, nervous system, and spirit so that I may be healed and strengthened".

Whilst placing this request, imagine swirling colours of pale blue and pale indigo flowing within you as the healing is taking place. When you feel much better, or notice a difference, (usually 2 mins.) command that the colours are ceasing to flow, and place a sincere thankyou to Archangel Chamuel, Fairy Queen Aerielle, and the plant devas of Chamomile.

When placing chamomile in the garden, request:

"Archangel Chamuel, Fairy Queen Aerielle, and plant deva of Chamomile, please allow your spiritual healing energies through Chamomile flow, to dispel hurt, anger, static emotions, and stagnancy from this garden, and to help the healing process of the ground, air, water, birds, animals, insects, plants, and my family. Thank-you."

A pale blue crystal may be placed next to the Chamomile plant to support it, and strengthen the healing processes.

You may also place fresh chamomile flowers in a bowl of water, or burn organic chamomile oil in a burner in the home to help clear the energies and to calm and balance, and say the affirmation.

Affirmation: "My whole being is now being soothed, calmed, and strengthened."

COMPOSITAE HERBS

CHICORY—(Cichorium intybus)

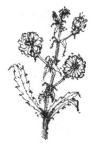

Part Used: Flower, whole plant.

Flower: Blue daisy flower

Actions: Cholagogue, digestive, diuretic, liver & Gallbladder tonic

Indications: Chicory aids digestion, and is a tonic to the liver, gallbladder, and spleen. It promotes bile production, helping us to digest fats. As a liver tonic it may aid in cholesterol and gallstones. The fresh flowers and leaves can be used in salads, and the root roasted for a coffee substitute drink.

ANGEL: **Archangel Samuel**

FAIRY: **Queen Chisarka**

WORD: **Accepting love**

Uses: Chicory uses the blue rays of a distant spiritual planet to help dispel anger, jealousy, loneliness and vindictiveness. It helps clear these emotions from the liver so that the heart can accept, and then give, happiness, love and praise. Its blue flowers reach above the other herbs towards the sky. It also raises us up from the negative emotions. Chicory gently tones up the liver and digestive enzymes to work more efficiently, cleaning out little grey matter over these areas which may cause sluggishness. Chicory when planted or dug into the earth helps to gently purify the ground, clears any hatred, and brings the blue healing energy in. This allows better uptake of nourishment for the other plants so they can grow stronger, and also clear the way for the nurturing fairies to come in to help the plants.

COLOUR: Chicory vibrates to a light blue and pale light lemon energy.

CHICORY

Chicory has beautiful spiritual energies, sent to it from a far off spiritual planet and galaxy.

By cleansing the liver and gallbladder it can gently release stuck heavy energies (from past lives) which are not needed now, as they are stale and old. Using Chicory, and then Calendula afterwards, will help clear, and then heal, these energies. This is why the chicory flower essence is helpful when people feel stuck, angry, hurt, jilted, abused, ignored, or unloved. It is often the reason why the flower essence can also help with the emotions of hyperactive children, two year old temper tantrums, sibling rivalry, or rivalry between pets, animals, and birds. Also used for PMT, puberty, and menopause when the emotions feel unbalanced due to hormonal changes.

When using chicory as an herb tea, using the flowers in a salad, or just sitting next to the plant, request:

"Archangel Samuel, Fairy Queen Chisarka, and plant devas of Chicory, please allow your spiritual energies assigned to Chicory, to flow into my body, mind and spirit, to calm the emotions held in my liver, gallbladder, and body, from this life and all past lives so I may feel happier and calmer, and be healed. Thank-you".

Think of swirls of pale light blue, and pale lemon yellow flowing into your body, especially the liver and gallbladder. When you feel lighter, or calmer, (2-3 mins.) command that the colours cease their flow, and place a sincere thank-you to Archangel Samuel, Fairy Queen Chisarka, and the plant devas of Chicory.

When planting Chicory in the garden or in a pot, place a request: "Archangel Samuel, Fairy Queen Chisarka, and plant devas of Chicory, please allow your spiritual energies through chicory, flow into my garden, into the ground, water, air, and the earth's crystal grid, to heal and cleanse all the stuck and stagnant emotions and energies from this life and past lives. May the healing, cleansing and balancing take place for the good of all. Thank-you."

A pale light blue and a pale lemon crystal may be placed next to Chicory to speed up the clearing and healing processes.

Affirmation: "I release stagnant and stuck emotions held in, from this life and past lives, so that my crystal grid, liver and gallbladder can be cleansed and balanced."

COMPOSITAE FAMILY

DANDELION—(Taraxacum officinale)

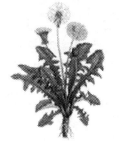

Part Used: Roots, leaves

Flower: Yellow daisy

Actions: Diuretic, digestive, liver tonic, gallbladder tonic

Indications: Dandelion is a good source of potassium, so, it can be useful as a diuretic for fluid retention. As a liver tonic it is used in formulas for weight loss, gallstones, cholesterol, jaundice, bloating, and congestion of the liver and gallbladder. It also aids digestion of fats and carbohydrates, so may help with midriff weight gain and bloating. With Berberis and other liver herbs it aids dissolving of gallstones.

ANGEL: **Archangel Metatron and his helpers.**

FAIRY: **King Letophile**

WORD: **Detoxer**

Uses: Energy is channeled through Dandelion from outside the solar system, via the sun to energize the earth and all of us. It is a golden energy, with gold and silver sparkles within it, from Archangel Metatron, to cleanse and strengthen us, and the earth. With this energy's seemingly magical powers to cleanse, many plant devas, earth and sun devas, and fairies come forward to work with Dandelion in the garden. Being high in potassium, it now allows electrical changes to take place in the body and earth, to renew systems and pathways and enzymes. Dandelion can also help cleanse the outer bodies and seal off cracks in the aura with its gold and silver sparkling energy. Notice that the flowers face towards the sun, and track's the sun's rays. At the end of winter, and the beginning of spring, they cover hills and paddocks to bring this revitalizing energy to Earth. Fresh Dandelion leaf tea gently helps the whole body, whilst the Dandelion root tea gets in deeper, to flush out toxins, and cleanse.

COLOUR: Dandelion radiates a vibrant gold energy with gold and silver sparkles within it.

DANDELION

Dandelion, with its high content of nutrients, especially potassium, has an affinity with water, so cleanses, re-oxygenates, and purifies the water in our body. By cleansing the water channels in the ground, between the roots of plants, trees and shrubs, the energies, nutrients, and oxygen, can be better utilized by the plants. It also helps to flush out deep seated, angry and jealous hurts, in the ground even from past lives. Many of our own stored and stagnant hurts and griefs, are held in the liver, and it's the liver which cleanses the blood so helping other organs and pathways in the body. Whilst drinking Dandelion tea, or eating the leaves or flowers in a salad, request:

"Archangel Metatron, Fairy King Letophile, and plant devas of Dandelion, please allow your spiritual energies, and the energies of the sun and the solar system, assigned to Dandelion, flow within me, to cleanse, detox, and purify stagnant hurts, and emotions in my body and aura. Also to unblock my crystal grid, purify my blood and strengthen my whole body."

Whilst placing this request, think of vibrant, gold energy with gold and silver sparkles in it, flowing into your whole being and aura. When you feel a difference, (2-3 mins.) command that the colour is ceasing it's flow, and then place a sincere thank-you to Archangel Metatron, Fairy King Letophile, and the plant devas of Dandelion.

When placing the Dandelion plant in the garden, request:

"Archangel Metatron, Fairy King Letophile, and plant devas of Dandelion, please allow your spiritual energies and the spiritual energies of the sun and the solar system flow into my garden, and into the ground, to cleanse, purify, revitalize, and oxygenate the water, the crystals, and the crystal grid of my garden. Please bring the fairies, gnomes, elves, sprites, and deva back to nurture, heal, and tend to all the plants, bird, insects, and animals, and to help mother nature. Thank-you."

A crystal of sparkling yellow or a white quartz crystal may be placed next to Dandelion to help the healing process.

Affirmation: I now release and cleanse all stagnant hurt, grief and anger held in my liver and body, so I may be healed and made whole and well.

LABIATAE HERBS

LAVENDER—(Lavandula officinalis)

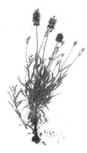

Part Used: Flowers, leaves

Flower: Whirls of tiny lilac tubular flowers

Actions: Carminative, antispasmodic, stomachic, antiseptic, mild antidepressant

Indications: Lavender is a gentle, strengthening tonic to the nervous system. Therefore it is useful with headaches, insomnia, anxiety, nervousness, and nervous debility and exhaustion. For depression it combines well with Rosemary. Externally it soothes aches, sprains, and sore muscles. Lavender is an antiseptic, and an insect repellent. A tea from the leaves can gently aid digestion.

ANGEL: **Archangel Gabriel**

FAIRY: **Queen Lelitha**

WORD: **Self Heal**

Uses: Lavender comes from a gentle far away planet to help with children, the elderly, animals, and especially the fearful. The lavender flowers emit Ray 7, one of the highest but most gentle healing rays. That is why it is particularly good for burns, and can even heal burns from past lives. It will seep through the layers of the skin to heal the matrix of the skin and subtle bodies, where burns have left a block. By gently releasing the memory of burns, fear, anxiety, and intrepidations, and allowing them to waft away, enables a person to move forward and try new ventures. Previously they may have seemed overwhelming. That is why it is beneficial to place Lavender on a baby's pillow every night to clear some of the past, and help them try new things in the future. Especially calming for earth birth-signs, when feeling boxed in or fearful of any changes. (or any of us)

COLOUR: Lavender emits a beautiful violet energy. The colour can transpose from the material into a higher, more spiritual vibration.

LAVENDER

Although Lavender is soothing and calming, it can also be a link breaker, by bringing in one of the highest and strongest Archangels to watch over, and protect us. Archangel Gabriel loves working with Lavender, and will stand no nonsense. Using organic Lavender oil, or crushed, fresh leaves and flowers in the house, will dispel dark clouds, strange aromas, and stubborn energies which are not shifting. Use Lavender for a week to break with the past, then a week of sage to tune to higher knowledge, and then a week of fresh calendula flowers to bring in the higher energies of joy and vitality from the sun and the solar system.

The Fairy Queen Lelitha is one of the highest, most nurturing of the Fairies and loves coming to our aid (especially the elderly, the gentle, and babies) so we can be stronger, calmer and less fearful. Birds, butterflies, insects, dragonflies, and smaller wildlife love her, as she darts around the garden to see if anyone is in need of her energies. We can drink Lavender tea, have a bath with organic oil or fresh leaves, rub the oil on our body, or place a drop on our pillow. The crushed leaves and flowers can be strewn around the house and in cupboards Whilst doing this or drinking the tea, request:

"Archangel Gabriel, Fairy Queen Lelitha, and the plant devas of Lavender, please allow your gentle spiritual energies through Lavender flow within me, to nurture, soothe, and strengthen my whole being, my aura and my spirit".

Imagine swirls of medium violet colour flowing around you, and in you, as you place this request. Once you feel the difference, command that the colour ceases and place a sincere thank-you to Archangel Gabriel, Fairy Queen Lelitha, and the plant deva of Lavender.

When placing Lavender in your garden, especially in any areas of land that has been burnt, or had bushfires, request:

"Archangel Gabriel, Fairy Queen Lelitha, plant Deva of Lavender, please soothe, calm, and heal this whole garden area, (or paddock or hillside) so that its crystal energy grid can be renewed, strengthened, and nurtured. Then bring the plant devas, spirits, sprites, and fairies back, to look after the plants, flowers, and wildlife. Thank-you."

Place a purple crystal or a white quartz crystal beside the Lavender plant to support it, and speed up the healing processes in that area.

Affirmation: "I release all dark clouds, strange aromas, and stubborn energies which are blocking me, so I may be nurtured, strengthened and healed."

LABIATAE HERBS

LEMON BALM – (Melissa offinalis)

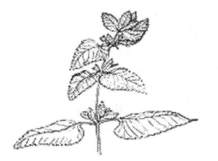

Part Used: Leaves

Flower: Tiny blue/white clusters

Actions: Carminative, antispasmodic, diaphoretic, antidepressive, hypotensive

Indications: Lemon balm is in the mint family so is helpful for upset tummies, dyspepsia, flatulence, and colic. It is excellent for bloating, and for calming nerves, especially when premenstrual. As it is slightly calming, it soothes anxiety, nervousness and PMT. Like mint it can also be used for colds and 'flu.

ANGEL: **Archangel Oriel**

FAIRY: **Queen Aurora**

WORD: **Calming**

Uses: Lemon Balm is high in magnesium, including a high frequency magnesium, so it can calm the physical body as well as the mind and the emotions. Lemon Balm has an aromatic scent which, when placed in the house, sends energies out to soothe and calm. Sprigs of the fresh herb can be placed over a baby's crib for Archangel Oriel and Queen Aurora to protect on a physical and spiritual level. The herb also repels insects. Lemon Balm calms the tummy and flows into the nerve endings of the stomach, going through the rest of the body and up into the brain, to calm the emotions. It works wonderfully well as a homoeopathic, or used as an oil. It has been used by the ancients in temples and healing centres, as a balm or ointment placed on the chakras, to calm old grief, shock, and unsettled emotions. This herb can also dispel subtle draining energies.

COLOUR: Lemon Balm vibrates a colour of pure white with pale blue.

LEMON BALM

Lemon Balm, belongs to the mint family, but has a gentle, spiritual crystal pattern which is arranged in such a way, as to take us up in to a higher mental state. It brings in soothing nurturing angels to heal our static emotions and this takes us, ever so slightly, above the emotions, so we can be more objective and understanding. The tea is very good for children, to calm and soothe them after school. It is also helpful for everyone, in this time of great change, and disorientation. Lemon Balm has a delightful lemon/mint flavour.

When drinking the tea or placing Lemon Balm in the bath, request:

"Archangel Oriel, Fairy Queen Aurora, and plant deva of Lemon Balm, please allow your spiritual energies flowing through Lemon Balm and its crystal patterns, flow within my body to calm, soothe and nurture my whole being as well as my crystal grid".

As you place this request, think of swirls of bright white and pale blue flowing within your whole being. When you feel the difference, (2-3 mins.), command, that the colours cease flowing, and then place a sincere thank-you, to Archangel Oriel, Fairy Queen Aurora, and the plant deva of Lemon Balm.

When growing Lemon Balm in the garden, notice how all the dragonflies, bees, butterflies and insects, swarm over to the plant and its flowers, so they can feel the beautiful calming, nurturing energies of the fairies and plant devas of Lemon Balm. Sit next to Lemon Balm and request:

"Archangel Oriel, Fairy Queen Aurora, and plant deva of Lemon Balm, please flow your spiritual energies through Lemon Balm, into this garden, to soothe, nurture, and heal the atmosphere, plants, fairies, sprites, birds, insects, and animals in my garden. Please remove the shock, trauma, and grief that has been caused by the toxins and chemicals, from the past, and allow the finer spiritual grid of the earth to be healed. Thank-you."

A pale blue, or blue and white crystal may be placed next to the Lemon Balm to enhance the nurturing, healing, processes.

Affirmation: "My digestion, nerves and whole being are now being soothed and calmed by the Lemon Balm."

LABIATAE HERBS

PEPPERMINT—(Mentha piperita)

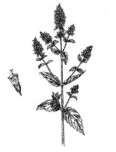

Part Used: leaves

Flower: small purple clusters

Actions: Antispasmodic, carminative, stomachic, antiseptic, diaphoretic, digestive.

Indications: Peppermint is taken for digestive problems such as indigestion, nausea, flatulence, colic, and travel sickness. It is also used for colds, 'flu, and catarrh. Peppermint gently calms the nerves, and cools overheated conditions. The oil rubbed on our temples with lavender oil helps headaches and migraines. Place sprigs of fresh mint over babies, and children's bed heads to repel insects, especially mosquitoes. Place fresh mint near doors and windows to repel insects.

ANGEL: **Archangel Sophiel**

FAIRY: **Queen Philipa**

WORD: **Stimulating**

Uses: Peppermint gently stimulates the cells, increasing their vitality and energy. This increase of energy can expel stagnant matter, uplifting the person so they can feel stronger, happier, and more complete. It helps clear out stagnancies in the ground, and to rid it of parasites, dank earth and rubbish, so that the earthworms, fairies and elves can come back to the garden. This creates a way for other herbs to come in and restore fertility and nourishment to the soil. The essential oils in the peppermint plant can uplift a dank house, and remove heaviness, and tiredness. The oils in Peppermint can cleanse some of our lower chakras, to help us see and think more clearly. (cleaning out the cobwebs) Peppermint also brings in a certain sense of excitement, refreshing the air, and so allowing changes to come in.

COLOUR: Peppermint vibrates a light lime green colour.

PEPPERMINT

Light lime green is refreshing, cooling, soothing and cleansing (think of a rain forest). Peppermint cools slightly inflamed conditions, such as excess heat in the body, and calms fractious nerve endings in the tummy, helping to expel wind. By slightly raising the energy of the cells and cleansing away the old cobwebs, peppermint can bring fresh, new energy in, lifting us gently above our thoughts. This removes the grey clouds, raising us above the solar plexus bringing in renewal, rebirth, vitality and freshness, thus creating a pathway for new beginnings. The vitality allows us to look at new ways of dealing with situations, and looking at ourselves. Following with sage tea will bring us up into the higher mind, to know which direction to follow, see the new doorways opening, and decide which one to choose. Sage and Peppermint together create a sense of positivity, strength and direction, as we move out of the cobwebs of heaviness and indecision. When drinking or eating organic peppermint request:

"Archangel Sophiel, Fairy Queen Philipa, plant deva of Peppermint, please allow your spiritual, revitalizing, energies to Peppermint to flow into my cells to uplift, revitalize, and re-energize my whole being".

Think of the light lime green flowing into your body, revitalizing and energizing. Then place a sincere thank-you to Archangel Sophiel, Fairy Queen Philipa, and the plant deva of Peppermint, and cease the flow of light lime green.

Remember how peppermints tingle in our mouth? When planting peppermint think of this tingling affect, refreshing, and renewing the ground and removing dank energies, moulds, and insects which are destroying the plants roots, harming them. Think of the tingling, also sparking up the energy pathways under the ground. By growing peppermint, digging it into the ground, or spraying the ground with peppermint tea, this will allow the good organisms to come in with the plant devas to also vitalize and cleanse the ground. Request: "Archangel Sophiel, Fairy Queen Philipa, and plant deva of Peppermint please allow your spiritual energies flowing through Peppermint, flow into the ground to remove stagnant darkness, dank matter, moulds, clouds, and heaviness. Please cleanse, renew, and revitalize the energy pathways that surround peppermint so that the fairies, elves, and plant devas can come in to continue the healing."

Place a light green crystal next to the Peppermint to support the healing.

Affirmation: "My whole being is now becoming refreshed, revitalised, energised, and uplifted."

LABIATAE HERBS

ROSEMARY–(Rosmarinus officinalis.)

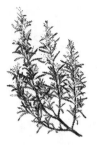

Part Used: leaves

Flower: clusters of small blue/purple flowers

Actions: Digestive, carminative, antiseptic antispasmodic, anti-depressive, anti-parasitic

Indications: Rosemary aids circulation, so is excellent for poor memory, chronic fatigue, sluggish blood flow, low blood pressure, cold hands and feet, and hair loss. It stimulates and aids the digestion, especially to digest fats and proteins. (eg. roast lamb with rosemary) It is helpful for flatulence and dyspepsia. The herb also helps in depression especially with wild oats tea, even where there is debility and poor circulation. Externally it stimulates the hair follicles to help new hair growth. Good for studying, and helping our memory. (not to be taken in pregnancy or with high blood pressure.)

ANGEL: **Archangel Zadkiel**

FAIRY: **Queen Marella**

WORD: **Energising**

Uses: Rosemary herb has an abundance of essential oils, potassium, and other nutrients which increase blood flow, memory and circulation. It stimulates the body to pull us up into the higher chakras, and into the higher mind. This increases the pathways between the right and left brain, to stimulate old creative memories, thoughts and abilities, which have been hidden. Rosemary helps the spiritual and material mind to work together, for painting and writing, by strengthening thought processes and understanding. It also clears creative blocks held in from the past. Rosemary helps the earth to remember joy from the past. It attracts lots of fairies, goblins, and elves which strengthen the roots of plants, and so increase the nourishment to plants to fortify them. Rosemary is strengthening, by giving fortitude and stamina, so the tea is good for chronic fatigue, or if feeling worn out, on a spiritual or physical level.

COLOUR: Rosemary's energies vibrate to a light bright orange colour.

ROSEMARY

Rosemary is one of the kings of herbs. It helps to activate the mind, including the higher minds, that's why it is good for memory, and chronic fatigue. It sends the blood running through the muscles and joints up into the brain. Along with sage, rosemary was used by monks, and temples, to awaken the higher mind and the higher chakras. This awakens the memories and the knowledge of past abilities which have been clouded over. Also good for remembering music, poetry, writing, mathematics, and skills we once had as teachers in past lives, other dimensions, and Atlantis. Rosemary is always used on remembrance day. It was added to flower posies, given to loved ones, to mean please remember me.

The herb is good for stagnant or slow moving conditions, as it pushes the nutrients and energy around the body to nourish the cells and organs. It then flows through the connecting pathways to the other bodies and meridians, and to the aura. Do an aura cleanse whilst drinking this tea. (visualize white light enveloping the aura, cleansing it or use your hands 4" away from the body, starting at the head down to the toes and then back up to the head to seal off all cracks in the aura). Even though its flowers are blue/violet, Rosemary resonates to the light orange on a mental, physical, and vitality level. So when drinking Rosemary tea, you can think of the light bright orange flooding into all of your cells to energize, vitalize, and uplift, and request:

"Archangel Zadkiel, Fairy Queen Marella, and plant deva of Rosemary, please allow your spiritual energies through Rosemary flow into me, to energize and vitalize all my cells, circulation, memory, and my whole being, from my toes up to my head and into my aura."

When you can feel the changes, command that the colour is ceasing, and place a sincere thank-you to Archangel Zadkiel, Fairy Queen Marella, and plant deva of Rosemary. When planting Rosemary in the garden, request":

"Archangel Zadkiel, Fairy Queen Marella, and plant deva of Rosemary, please allow your spiritual energies to flow through Rosemary from the stars into the ground, to renew, refresh, revitalize and energize all the pathways in the ground. Let nourishment flow out to the plants, insects, birds, and wildlife so they can enjoy these new spiritual energies coming in, thank-you."

You may place a light orange crystal next to the Rosemary plant to enhance the healing.

Affirmation: "My whole being is now being refreshed, revitalized, and energized on all levels."

LABIATAE HERBS

SAGE—(Salvia officinalis)

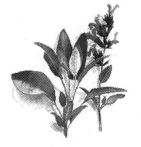

Part Used: Leaves

Flowers: Red, and bluish/purple flowers.

Actions: Antiseptic, antihydrotic, carminative, antibacterial

Indications: Sage is used for all inflammations of the mouth, throat, tonsils, and gums especially for gingivitis, sore throats, laryngitis, mouth ulcers, pharyngitis, and colds and 'flu. Sage often helps to dry up profuse sweating, especially in menopause. It can be used for memory, focus and energy. Avoid Sage during lactation as it can dry up milk supplies.

ANGEL: **Archangel Chakriel**

FAIRY: **King Wultter**

WORD: **Knowing**

Uses: Sage is highly antiseptic, so reduces inflammations of the respiratory tract. It especially helps the throat chakra, which has an affinity with the mind chakra. (speaking your mind). Sage will help us to speak our truth, that is why it is used to clear out houses, to allow only the energies of truth to come in. Sage can also clear the aura of what is not our own (false attachments). It also helps to bring the bodies into alignment, and so remove confusing energies, whether from the past or the present. One drop of sage oil can clear out a house of tired or unethical energies. After sage, use lemon oil to fill up the space left behind, to keep it clear and fresh, and vibrating at a higher wavelength.

COLOUR: Sage emits energies of a subtle colour of light dark red, then light blue.

SAGE

Sage is another master herb. Some Sage flowers are a brilliant red, like the fire element, and others are a blue/violet colour, like the other Labiatae family plants. Sage is a cooling herb to the physical body. However, it also has a red energy to the fire element,—to" burn out" dark, unwanted, energies out of the house, the atmosphere, and those which envelop the throat and the mind. Sage quickly brings in the higher mind to work with the normal material mind, so that our spiritual commands of clearing and protection will work more efficiently. The positive energies of Mercury, and the positive energies of Venus (which are close to the earth so affect us greatly), both work through sage, helping us to be aligned, and so giving us better clarity and focus. That is why Sage tea is good to take for exams, and with meditation and cleansing. It helps to cut through any confusion and haze, to see more clearly, especially when others only want us to be confused.

The light blue in Sage helps to balance us, and to bring in the subtle communication of the higher mind through the throat chakra, whilst the red in Sage gives strength, vitality and protection. When drinking Sage tea or cooking with fresh Sage, request:

"Archangel Chakriel, Fairy King Wultter, plant deva of Sage, please allow your spiritual energies through sage, to the light red, flow within me and burn out unwanted microbes, clouds, and all that is not my own. (1-2 min.) Then flow within me the subtle Sage energies to the light blue for better communication, with calmness, and clarity".

Whilst requesting, think of swirls of light blue and light dark red enveloping your whole being. Then when you feel the change, place a sincere thank-you to Archangel Chakriel, Fairy King Wultter and the plant devas of Sage.

When planting Sage in the garden, place a request:

"Archangel Chakriel, Fairy King Wultter, and plant devas of Sage, may your spiritual energies, and the positive energies of Mercury and Venus, to Sage, flow into the garden and ground to burn out dark or dank unwanted toxins, clouds, or chemicals so that the plants and ground can be renewed, revitalized, and strengthened. Thankyou".

You may place a light blue crystal and a light dark red crystal next to the Sage plant to enhance the healing process.

Affirmation: "My whole being is now being cleansed of all that is not my own, so that I can be strengthened, have clarity, and be protected."

LABIATAE HERBS

THYME—(Thymus vulgaris)

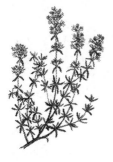

Part Used: Leaves

Flower: small bluish purple clusters

Actions: Antimicrobial, carminative

Indications: Thyme is used for sore throats, laryngitis, tonsillitis, bronchitis, coughs, and whooping cough. It is used to expel worms. Externally it is used as an antiseptic for infected wounds and funghal infections. Thyme tincture was used in hospitals until recently, as a potent antiseptic to sterilize floors.

ANGEL: **Archangel Fadkiel**

FAIRY: **King Tanuk and Queen Aurora**

WORD: **Eliminator**

Uses: Thyme contains energies of the moon and the constellations, to help remove worms, parasites, and spiritual tags of an annoying and draining nature. Thyme can heal very ancient illnesses of old structure and formation, especially of Greek and Egyptian origins, from past lives. It unblocks the grid or prism of the old bacteria or bug, for it to be rendered useless. Some energies of the moon have affected us adversely for a very long time, so may be hard to shift. Thyme can undo any energy matrix of this nature, and nullify it. Sage tea can then be taken after Thyme, to purify the surrounding area affected, and Rosemary next, to energize and vitalize.

COLOUR: Thymes energies vibrate a swirl of light yellow, and a violet/purple colour.

THYME

Thyme contains within it, amazing qualities of positive Pluto, positive Uranus, and positive moon energies. These energies, combined with its crystal structure, and plant devas, enables Thyme to delve in deeply, to remove parasites, worms and funghi. They act on a physical level as well as a spiritual level, working on stubborn, blocking formulas that have been held within us, for many lifetimes. The energies of the planets being utilized now by Archangel Fadkiel, Fairy King Tanuk and Queen Aurora, can go back, to Egyptian and Mesopotamian times to unlock these blockages, and remove and release them gently. This is because Archangel Fadkiel, fairy King Tanuk, and fairy Queen Aurora, were assigned to Earth during those eras, so understand the keys and symbols needed to unlock, and undo, the formulas held in from those times. They have kindly offered to come in and help us now. So if you are feeling drained, exhausted or heavy, use fresh Thyme in your cooking and drink Thyme tea with a little honey and request:

"Archangel Fadkiel, Fairy King Tanuk, Fairy Queen Aurora, and plant deva of Thyme, please allow your spiritual energies through Thyme, flow within me to cleanse my whole body and grid of parasites, worms, funghi, and formulae, held in from long ago, and ages past. Let my whole being be unblocked, purified, cleansed and cleared, so my spiritual energies may again flow through my crystal grid, to heal and strengthen my whole being".

With the request, imagine swirls of light yellow and medium violet flowing within your body until you feel the changes. Then command that the colours cease flowing, and place a sincere thank-you to Archangel Fadkiel, Fairy King Tanuk, Queen Aurora, and the plant devas of Thyme for helping.

When planting Thyme in the garden request:

"Archangel Fadkiel, Fairy King Tanuk, Fairy Queen Aurora, plant deva of Thyme, please allow your spiritual energies to Pluto, Uranus and the moon, flow through Thyme into my garden to awaken the plant and ground gnomes, spirits, elves and fairies to cleanse the earth's crystal grid. May they heal and vitalize the earth, water and air, so that the insects, butterflies, and dragonflies can live there and tend the plants and flowers.

A crystal of light yellow or violet purple can be placed next to the Thyme plant to help the healing processes.

Affirmation: "My whole being is releasing parasites and formulas from times past so that I can now be strengthened and vitalized."

LILIACEA HERBS

GARLIC – (Allium sativum)

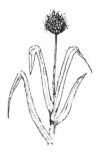

Part Used: bulb

Flower: Umbel of small white flowers

Actions: Bacteriostatic, decongestant, antiseptic, digestive, anthelmintic antibacterial.

Indications: Garlic is high in natural sulphur compounds, which help boost the immune system. It breaks up congestion, and is antibacterial, so helps overcome colds and 'flu. It is antiseptic and antipyrutic, so can clear up pus in wounds, cysts and boils. As it is able to lower cholesterol, it may aid the body's processes in lowering blood pressure (with other herbs). Garlic dispels worms, parasites and scabies. A tea of fresh crushed garlic, grated ginger, hot water and honey is excellent for overcoming colds and 'flu quickly, especially with a pinch of cayenne.

ANGEL: **Archangel Anturian**

FAIRY: **King Solaris**

WORD: **Antiseptic**

Uses: Garlic is now drawing on the energies of Mars and the Sun, due to its sulphur attributes. It therefore purifies our body, and the earth, ridding both of parasites, old pus, stagnant waters, and accumulated rubbish, where anaerobic micro-organisms grow, multiply and fester. It also clears stagnant bogs in the ground. Garlic helps with deep, putrid, stagnant energies, wounds, emotions and feelings. By causing the anaerobic organisms to die off, the good organisms, which are vital for life, can multiply and grow. This allows life-sustaining oxygen to come in for cell renewal, wound healing and repair.

COLOUR: The Garlic plant vibrates a bright golden yellow colour.

GARLIC

Garlic, through its sulphur compounds, and the strong active energies of Mars and the Sun, is unstoppable at burning out stubborn anaerobic organisms, (not only physically but also spiritually) which cause putrid, stagnant situations. Garlic helps them to dissolve or move out, by giving them an active shove, making way for oxygen and healing energies to come in and reclaim the space left behind. This is especially important if it there is an old block on your crystal grid causing ill health. Garlic is also a magical herb used by the ancients, for its energies and properties, which create a cardinal cross, are so very powerful at dispelling dark formulas and blocked energies.

Whilst eating or cooking fresh garlic, or making a tea of garlic, lemon and honey, imagine the bright golden yellow colour, flowing within you and request:

"Archangel Anturian, Fairy King Solaris and plant devas of Garlic, please allow your positive spiritual energies through Garlic, flow within me to burn out all parasites, viruses, dross, and stagnant or putrid energies in my being. May I be strengthened, cleansed, oxygenated, and healed."

When you can feel the change, place a sincere thank-you to Archangel Anturian, Fairy King Solaris and the plant devas of Garlic.

When placing garlic in the garden, think of golden yellow flowing into the ground and place the request:

"Archangel Anturian, Fairy King Solaris, and plant devas of Garlic please allow your spiritual energies to flow into this garden to remove all dank, dark, and stagnant water, air, earth, or conditions. Then oxygen, and nutrients can strengthen and heal all the plants, the ground, the air, and the earth's grid, to bring back the fairies, elves, butterflies, plant devas and insects, thank-you."

A bright yellow crystal can be placed next to Garlic to enhance the healing process.

Affirmation: "My whole being is now being cleansed, purified, and oxygenated so healing can begin."

ROSACEA HERBS

RASPBERRY—(Rubus idaeus)

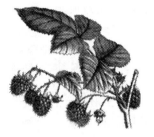

Part Used: Leaf

Flower: small white flower

Actions: Astringent, tonic, nutritive,

Indications: Raspberry leaf strengthens and tones the cells of the uterus and womb, thus aiding effective contractions in labour. Drink the tea in the last trimester. As an astringent, it can be helpful in diarrhoea, mouth ulcers and bleeding gums. The fruit is high in vitamin C which aids the uptake and utilization of iron, and the leaves are high in iron and folic acid, so helps overcome anaemia aiding oxygenation of the whole body.

ANGEL: **Archangel Uriel**

FAIRY: **Queen Anaphiel**

WORD: **Blood Tonic**

Uses: Raspberry contains energies of Venus and Mars. Raspberry leaf has a toning, strengthening effect, especially on the fibres of muscle, sinew, the ethereal matrix and the inner bodies. Being high in vitamin C, it helps these structures because vitamin C helps the body to make collagen. The blood red juice strengthens the blood, allowing it to carry nutrients to the rest of the body. Raspberry contains within it old Celtic healing energies which are very strong, tenacious and fortifying. Raspberry has placed within its structure, Celtic symbols for sustaining energies to strengthen the baby (hence for pregnant women) on many levels. Raspberry also brings in symbols from an outer planet for fortifying the body.

COLOUR: Raspberry vibrates to ruby red for fortifying, and to forest green for the old Celtic nourishment and sustenance.

RASPBERRY

Because Raspberry leaf tones the cells, and muscles of the uterus, helping the process of conception, (a most important and powerful time), this plant is lovingly watched over by Archangel Uriel and Fairy Queen Anaphiel. Everything must be perfect for the new soul coming in. Raspberry's energies of Venus for balancing the body, and its Mars energies to growth, new beginnings, renewal and expansion, work together to aid conception on a physical and spiritual level. Other herbs can also combine with Raspberry at this time. Raspberry fruit with the positive Mars energies, nourishes and strengthens the blood, increases Iron, Vitamin C and nutrient uptake, as well as strengthens the arteries, and blood vessels of the mother and the baby.

When making Raspberry leaf tea from the fresh leaves visualize the ruby red energy flowing within your body, as you request:

"Archangel Uriel, Fairy Queen Anaphiel, plant devas of Raspberry, please allow your spiritual energies flowing through Raspberry, flow within me to strengthen, nourish, and fortify my blood, cells, circulation and whole being." After you feel the change, place a thankyou. (It can aid preparation for conception and labour.)

When placing Raspberry in a pot or in the garden, request:

"Archangel Uriel, Fairy Queen Anaphiel, and plant devas of Raspberry, please allow your spiritual energies to flow into the ground, to fortify, strengthen and nourish the water, air and ground. May the environment be enriched, to bring back the elves, pixies, fairies, gnomes and plant devas into the garden, to heal the Earth and its crystal grid. Thank-you."

You may place a ruby red crystal, and a green crystal next to the raspberry plant to enhance the healing processes.

Affirmation: "My whole being is now being nourished, fortified, and strengthened."

UMBELLIFERAE HERBS

DILL —(Anethum graveolens)

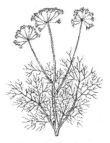

Part Used: seeds

Flower: umbels of small yellow flowers

Actions: Diuretic, carminative, galactagogue, antispasmodic.

Indications: Dill is used for flatulence, wind, colic, bad breath, and digestion, due to its aniseed type oils (aniseed is in the same herb family). Dill tea may help the milk to flow in lactating mothers. When the mother drinks the tea it flows through the milk to the baby to help relieve colic and digestive upsets in babies. Dill water is still popular for colic in babies.

ANGEL: **Archangel Suriel**

FAIRY: **King Favriel**

WORD: **Contentment**

Uses: Dill has aniseed type oils within it, to settle the stomach and expel wind ie: getting rid of something we can't stomach. Dill now uses the very subtle energies of an ethereal blue planet to dispel bad gas on many levels. The Dill plant when dug into the garden, will dispel bad gas pockets of fermenting energy, and hence allow water and nutrients to come in and saturate the soil with goodness. Sometimes different coloured gaseous energy cannot only settle in the stomach and intestines, but also in the aura, causing subtle energy changes and misalignments. Most of these changes we may not even notice. The planetary energies Dill brings in can help to dissolve these gases and remove the misalignment. The silvery light blue is very calming and subtle to babies, but they will feel it.

COLOUR: Dills energies vibrate a silvery light blue colour.

DILL

Because of its structure, Dill has a very fine, subtle, matrix and energy grid. This is why its properties are good for babies. It has gentle, soothing energies to calm the nerve endings, the stomach, the ethereal body, as well as calming nervous dispositions or traits carried over from past lives. Although very gentle and subtle, it works slowly, changing the wavelength of the agitated cells to a calming, peaceful, wavelength. Because of the oils in the leaves, it was used in the middle-ages and medieval times, to dispel bad gases, formulas, clouds, and bad gaseous smells. Some were of a spiritual nature, both in the body and in the house. Breastfeeding mothers can have Dill tea, and its qualities will flow to their baby, dispelling colic, wind, anxiety and nervousness.

Whilst drinking the tea, visualize a light silvery blue colour swirling around you, and in your body as you request:

"Archangel Suriel, Fairy Queen Favriel, and plant devas of Dill, please allow your spiritual energies from the silvery blue planet flow through Dill, and within me to soothe and calm my nervous system, stomach, and intestines, and to realign my whole being."

When you feel the difference within you, command that the colour ceases its flow, and place a sincere thankyou to Archangel Suriel, Fairy Queen Favriel and the plant deva of Dill."

Plant Dill in the garden because all the tiny butterflies, insects and fairies love its delicate nature and scent, and love to bathe in the silvery blue energies it radiates, soothing and healing them.

Place it in the garden or in a pot in the garden, and request:

"Archangel Suriel, Fairy Queen Favriel, and plant devas of Dill, please allow your spiritual energies, and those of the silvery blue planet to flow through Dill, into the ground, water, and air to soothe, and nurture the plants, insects, butterflies and animals so they may be healed and harmonized. Thank-you."

You may place a silvery blue crystal beside the Dill plant to strengthen the healing processes.

Affirmation: "My whole being is now being soothed, calmed, healed and re-aligned."

UMBELLIFERAE HERBS

FENNEL —(Foeniculum vulgare).

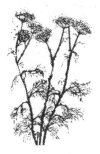

Part Used: Seed

Flower: large umbels of small yellow flowers

Actions: Antispasmodic, carminative, stomachic, galactogogue, aromatic, expectorant

Indications: Fennel, like Dill, aids in colic, wind, digestion, cramps, and bloating, by calming the tummy with its aniseed type properties. It may calm coughs and bronchitis, as it is mildly expectorant. Fennel also aids milk flow in lactating mothers. Because Fennel helps digestion, especially digestion of carbohydrates, the tea is helpful in a weight loss regime with other herbs.

ANGEL: **Archangel Zaniel**

FAIRY: **Queen Floriad**

WORD: **Dispeller**

Uses: Although much of Fennels energies come from the Sun, some comes from a sister planet of the Sun, and from positive Pluto. Its flower is a bright yellow umbel like the colour of the Sun. Fennel is stronger than Dill, with its properties purifying and dispelling bad gas, especially gaseous type formulas which have been around for eons. Remember in past ages, much knowledge was known of herb formulas and recipes. Think of the dark gases of bogs and marshes, and other planetary energies. If we can dispel some of these old stagnant energies, new energies from a higher level can come in now, to uplift and vitalize us. Fennel can undo some of the old energies of Vulcan and other planets which have affected us in the past and during many lifetimes. By dispelling all these formulas on many levels, it may help with weight loss and aid better flow of the bodily fluids and systems.

COLOUR: Fennel's energies vibrate a citrus green/ yellow colour.

FENNEL

Although having similar aniseed properties to Dill, Fennel has much stronger actions which dispel heavier and more resistant, gases and energies, especially of a physical nature. Many past life emotions and formulas are held in the liver, as well as in the murky rubbish in the intestines. This allows them to stick like bits of rubbery glue. Fennels properties, and the energies of Archangel Zaniel, Fairy Queen Floriad, and the positive energies of Pluto, are now ready to dissolve these formulas, and transmute them. Pluto has been recently unlocked by Archangel Zaniel to allow it to make the changes available to us. Drink small amounts of fresh fennel tea, visualizing a citrus green/yellow colour swirling within you and request:

"Archangel Zaniel, Fairy Queen Floriad, and plant devas of Fennel please allow your spiritual energies flowing through Fennel, flow within my whole being, to dispel old gases, gaseous formulas, and stagnant energies so changes can be made, and I can be strengthened."

When you feel the difference, place a sincere thank-you to Archangel Zaniel, Fairy Queen Floriad, and the plant devas of Fennel for coming forward now to help us.

When placing the Fennel plant in the garden request:

"Archangel Zaniel, Fairy Queen Floriad, plant devas of Fennel, please allow your energies to flow through Fennel, into the ground, water and air, to dispel any stagnant and gaseous energies. May this area be cleansed, cleared, and purified for the benefit of all the plants, fairies, insects, birds, butterflies and animals and for the earth's grid. Thankyou".

You may place a citrus green crystal next to the Fennel plant to enhance the cleansing and healing processes

Affirmation: All unwanted or stagnant energies are being dispelled from my being. I am now being cleansed and strengthened."

UMBELLIFERAE HERBS:

PARSLEY—(Petroselinum sativum)

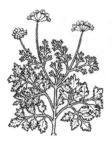

Part Used: leaves, seeds

Flower: umbels of small greenish/yellow flowers

Actions: Diuretic, emmenogogue, carminative.

Indications: Parsley is high in vitamin C, iron, silica, potassium, and some calcium and magnesium. It is a diuretic, so aids the removal of excess fluid, as well as dissolves crystals in the joints (like celery) in arthritis. Parsley also flushes out fluids through the kidneys and bladder. This helps overcome bladder retention, and flushes out the bacteria which aggravates cystitis. (Yarrow, another Umbelliferae herb, also helps) Parsley is a good, iron rich food to help in anaemia. Avoid large amounts of the juice in pregnancy.

ANGEL: **Archangel Savarone**

FAIRY: **Queen Favarelle & her helpers.**

WORD: **Releaser**

Uses: Parsley, like the other Umbelliferae plants (such as carrot, yarrow and celery), is a diuretic, therefore works through the kidneys to dispel fluid wastes. It draws some energies from the Sun, but also some positive energies from Saturn, to help flush out fears and blocks from the past. Because Parsley is high in lots of nutrients, the birds and the ground receive nourishment from them. Its roots can bring in the energies of the Sun and Saturn to break up stubborn rock hard blocks in the earth. This allows water to easily flow through the soils particles and nourish all growing things within the earth. The plant can be dug into the soil to help unblock old deposits of various types, either physical, spiritual, or ethereal, and cleanse the earths grid to allow it to be strengthened. Then the fairies, plant deva, gnomes, and elves can help heal the area.

COLOUR: Parsleys energies vibrates a bright green/yellow colour.

PARSLEY

Parsley has a strong concentration of minerals in its structure, so it can break up crystals in the kidneys and joints as does celery. It can be eaten raw in salads, as a tea, or in mixed juices, but must be used in small amounts so it is not too strong for the body.

The structure of Parsley, by being able to break up small crystals in the body and re-align them, helps to flush out fears held in the kidneys and bladder. Especially fears from past lives, concerning wars, conflict, and Viking raids, where the fear has stopped the kidneys from flushing out wastes. The fear (and sometimes dark shadows), has changed some of the structure of the minerals in the body thus causing the fluid retention, and altering the electrolyte balance. For releasing fear held in the kidneys, and releasing dark clouds or shadows causing blockages, place a request, as you visualize a bright yellow green swirling through your body.

"Archangel Savarone, Fairy Queen Favarelle with her pixies, and plant devas of Parsley, please allow your spiritual energies to flow within me to dispel fluids and wastes through my kidneys, bladder, joints, and whole being, so I may be strengthened."

When you can feel a change (2-5 mins.), place a sincere thank-you to Archangel Savarone, Fairy Queen Favarelle and the plant devas of Parsley.

When planting Parsley in the garden, notice its fresh cleansing aroma, and request:

"Archangel Savarone, Fairy Queen Favarelle and her pixies, and plant devas of Parsley, please allow your spiritual energies to flow into the ground, air, water, and the earth's crystal grid, to cleanse and purify them. May the fairies, pixies, gnomes, insects, butterflies and birds have fresh, clear, air, water, and earth to work in."

Place a bright yellow/ green crystal beside Parsley to help the processes, if you wish.

Affirmation:" My body is now being cleansed, detoxed, purified, and strengthened."

UMBELLIFERAE HERBS

YARROW—(Achillea millefolium)

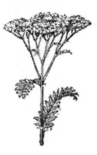

Part Used: leaves and flowers

Flower: Umbels of small white flowers

Actions: Diaphoretic, hypotensive, vulnerary, diuretic, antiseptic, hemostatic, and tonic

Indications: Yarrow may aid in lowering blood pressure by improving circulation and toning up the blood vessels. It aids in strengthening the lungs, so helps with more oxygenation throughout the body. Because it can help reduce fevers, Yarrow is often used in cold and sinus mixtures with elder and peppermint. It helps internally, and externally, to heal wounds. (one of my canaries was attacked by a large bird, and had a bad wound, but fresh yarrow tea via the beak and in his water healed it up beautifully). Yarrow is excellent for flushing out the bladder, so is needed in cystitis and fluid retention. Yarrow aids externally by healing leg ulcers, and soothing haemorrhoidal bleeding.

ANGEL: **Archangel Michael and his angels.**

FAIRY: **King Santonelle & Queen Florissa**

WORD: **Wound healer**

Uses: Yarrow has within it, energies of renewal, regrowth, reunification, and regeneration. It is able to stimulate new cell growth in bodily tissue, to heal old cuts and wounds internally and externally. It draws on the energies of Neptune and Jupiter, and another healing planet, to bring in new energies to the earth, to stimulate new growth from seeds, buds, twigs, and seemingly dormant wood and soil. It is beneficial to dig the Yarrow plant into compost heaps to revitalize the soil. Yarrow, on a spiritual level, can now slowly, repair and remove from past lives, old stagnant patterns causing blocks, pain, injury or disorders. This is especially so, from past lives of war, conflict, famine, starvation, or consumption.

COLOUR: Yarrow vibrates a swirl of bright white and light pink colours.

YARROW

Yarrow is a master healing herb and draws on the energies of positive Venus, positive Jupiter, and positive Neptune for our renewal, regrowth, and re-awakening. These energies are coming in at this time through Archangel Michael and his angels, especially to awaken our spiritual self-love, spiritual self-esteem, and self-nurturing. These have all been blocked of later times, greatly affecting our health and well-being. When we feel healthy, happy, and balanced, this positivity flows out to others and helps them to move forward too. Through Archangel Michaels love for us and Fairy Queen Florissa's gentle caring, Yarrow can flush out toxins and fluids, through the kidneys and bladder. It also flushes out fear, shock, and grief from wars, conflict and famine. The angels want to help us remove all these old energies which have been holding us back. Then they can bring in the new spiritual energies to help us progress on our spiritual pathway, to move forward with ease and grace, and to become who we want to become. For strengthening, healing and aligning your energies, and bodies, think of white and light pink, swirling through your body as you request:

"Archangel Michael, Fairy King Santonelle, Fairy Queen Florissa, and plant devas of Yarrow, please allow your spiritual energies flowing through Yarrow, flow within my whole being, to strengthen, balance, harmonize and heal all my bodies, cells, and spirit, as well as healing old wounds from the past."

When you feel the changes, (2-5 mins. or longer), place a sincere thank-you to Archangel Michael, Fairy King Santonelle, Fairy Queen Florissa and the plant devas of Yarrow.

When placing Yarrow in the garden, request:

"Archangel Michael, Fairy King Santonelle, and Fairy Queen Florissa, please allow your spiritual energies and the energies of positive Venus, Jupiter and Neptune, flow into my garden, to heal the water, earth, and air, and the Earth's crystal grid. Then the fairies, elves, sprites, and gnomes may attend to all the plants, insects, birds, and butterflies, as is needed for healing and awakening. Thankyou."

A crystal of pink quartz and a crystal of white quartz may be placed next to Yarrow to help the healing processes.

Affirmation: "I am being healed, cleansed and made whole and well again, so my spiritual energies may be awakened and increased."

HERBAL PREPARATIONS

1. **Herbal teas**—as infusions for flowers, leaves, seeds, stems.

   Use 1-2 teaspoons of chopped fresh herbs in a china or glass teapot, or coffee plunger. Pour boiling water over and steep for 10-15 minutes. Drink hot, or cold. Lemon, mint, ginger, honey or ice can be added. Or use a small tea infuser ball for just one cup.

2. **Herbal teas**—as decoctions for roots, bark, wood, seeds.

   Place 1-2 teaspoons of chopped fresh herbs with 1-2 cups of water, in a glass or stainless steel saucepan. Bring to the boil, and simmer 10-15 mins. Strain, and drink.

3. **Salads and cooking.**

   Add fresh herbs and/or their flowers to salads and cooking.

4. **Baths**

   Add fresh herbs or flowers, or herb tea, to your bath. eg. Lavender or chamomile to help sleep, fennel for slimming, yarrow and calendula to heal eczema or psoriasis, or sunburn.

5. **Compresses**

   For healing and drawing out pus, use linen, cotton, or gauze or cotton wool soaked in a warm herbal infusion, to place on the skin.

6. **Washes**

   Make an herb tea, let it cool, and wash skin, or eyes. Chamomile is great for soothing sunburn or sore eyes. Yarrow and calendula, for wounds and ulcers.

7. **Oils**

   Add fresh herbs to vegetable oils and leave 2-3 weeks for use in cooking & salads.

8. **Insect repellents**

   Sprigs of herbs, such as Lavender, Thyme, Rosemary and others, can be dried and placed into drawers and wardrobes to repel insects. Fresh mint placed over babies and children's beds, or above doorways can repel mosquitoes. Herb teas used as a wash around window sills or over kitchen benches repels ants.

There are also many other ways the fresh herbs can be used, to bring into your daily life.

EXPLANATIONS OF ACTIONS OF HERBS

Alterative: Blood purifying
Analgesic: pain relieving
Anodyne: reduces pain
Anthelmintic: expels worms
Antibacterial: acts against infective bacteria
Antifunghal: acts against funghal infection
Anithydrotic: reduces excessive sweating
Antimicrobial: acts against disease causing organisms
Antiinflamatory: reduces severity of inflamation
Antispasmodic: reduces spasms and cramps
Antidepressant: uplifts moods
Antirheumatic: eases rheumatic complaints
Astringent: causes tightening to reduce inflamation
Aromatic: having strong taste or smell
Bacteriostatic: reduces disease causing bacteria
Cardiac: acts as a tonic to the heart muscle
Carminative: eases flatulence, colic, and wind
Cholagogue: aids liver and gallbladder function
Diaphoretic: promotes sweating to reduce fever or infection
Digestive: aids better digestion
Diuretic: aids fluid excretion through the kidneys and bladder
Decongestant: reduces congestion so helps coughing
Expectorant: encourages expulsion of mucous from respiratory tract
Emmenogogue: promotes menstruation
Febrifuge: able to reduce fever
Galactogogue: promotes milk flow in lactating mothers
Hepatic: enhances liver function
Hypotensive: aids lowering of blood pressure naturally
Insecticidal: repels unwanted insects
Nervine: nervous system tonic
Nutritive: high in nutrients so is nourishing
Parasitic: aids expulsion of parasites
Rubifacient: brings heat to the skin

Sedative:	helps to induce sleep
Stimulant:	increases energy or stimulates a body's function
Stomachic:	promotes digestive activity of the stomach
Tonic:	nourishes body to restore better function
Vermifuge:	expels worms
Vulnerary:	helps wound healing

SOLAR RADIANCE

Wouldn't it be wonderful to start the day feeling as refreshed as if we'd been on a long walk through the rainforest?

For us to remain focused, clear, positive, energetic, and to feel more like our true selves, the keys to cleansing our auras, bodies, and houses are needed. Cleansing will also improve our awareness and communication with our guardian angels and spirit guides, helping us become that light unto the world. Many of us already utilize colour, sound, energies, music or bells to cleanse or protect our homes or ourselves. However the Beings of Light want this new knowledge to be given so each of us can be empowered, and utilize these energies for ourselves.

One of the nicest and most effective energies given to us by the Beings of Light, to use in our daily lives, is Solar Radiance, a sparkling gold energy from the universe. It is a beautiful cleansing, vitalizing, effective, but gentle, light with amazing properties. Solar Radiance radiates from our solar system to enliven and sustain all life forms on this planet.

Because our own thoughts and emotions, and those of others, build daily in the astral and emotional levels of our aura, bodies, and meridians, we get drained, tired and enveloped. Solar Radiance is the perfect light for us to cleanse with, each morning, to be refreshed, strengthened, and balanced. This helps us to know our own self, and have a calm, clear mind. However it is also more effective to cleanse our house or room first, to clear the air so to speak, before we then cleanse ourselves.

CLEANSING THE HOUSE WITH SOLAR RADIANCE

Sit quietly, relax, close your eyes and imagine a sparkling gold light flowing through the roof and into your whole house. (you don't need to see it, it will happen) So the Beings of Light know what you want the light to do, you must give it direction with your command, as you visualize or feel it is happening.

1. Command: "Solar Radiance is flowing and increasing into my house." (rpt.1-3 times until you feel it building.)

2. Command: "The Solar Radiance I have increased within my house is cleansing my house of all thought forms, emotional forms, dross, and all negative energies. The Solar Radiance is sending it all out into the universe to be dissolved." (rpt. 3-4 times)

When a change is felt the house has been cleansed, and the cleared space needs to be filled.

3. Request: "Beings of Light may Solar Radiance flow and increase within my house for harmony and balance." (or for happiness and upliftment.)—wait 1-2 mins., for the change.

4. So that this harmony and balance stays within the house request:

    "Beings of Light may the Solar Radiance flow around the outside of my house to build a golden shield of protection to repel all thought forms, emotional forms, dross and negative energies." After a couple of minutes, thank the Beings of Light for helping us.

CLEANSING YOUR AURA & BODIES

The steps to cleansing your body with Solar Radiance, is similar to cleansing your house. Sit quietly, and close your eyes:

1. Request to the Beings of Light: "May Solar Radiance flow into my aura, mental body, astral/emotional body, physical body, and meridians, cleansing them of all thought forms, emotional forms, dross, and negative energies. Solar Radiance is pushing them all out into the universe to be dissolved." (repeat until you feel the change)

2. Then request: "May Solar Radiance flow into my aura, mental body, astral/ emotional body, physical body and meridians, strengthening them and balancing them." (rpt.1-3 times).

    When you feel the change, place a thank-you to the Beings of Light who are here to help us.

    You may also use this request for "healing and upliftment," or "for energy and vitality" if you need it, or "for balance and a competent mind," if you have exams. You will know what you need on the day.

This exercise will balance you for the day, but can easily be repeated anytime during the day (or night) if you so need it, to help you feel stronger, more focused and able to think more clearly. However there are also many more quick commands you may do if needed. You can do them either after cleansing with the Solar Radiance, or you can just do them on their own to very quickly bring you into balance and focus. Balancing the bodies can be done as many times as you want during the day. (or night)

BALANCING THE BODIES

Thoughts build up in the Mental levels, and emotions build up in the Astral levels, including our fears, worries and illusions. We don't want them to stay with us all day, and make us feel lethargic, or be unable to think, or allow them to pull us down into the lower chakras. These commands are quick, and easy to do:

1. My mental mind and body is vibrating, flowing, and communicating up into
    . . . Mental level 7

2. My physical body is vibrating, and flowing up into
    . . . Physical level 7.

3. My astral/emotional body is vibrating, and flowing up into
    . . . Astral/Emotional level 7.

4. My mental, astral, physical, and spiritual body energies are flowing, combining and blending as one. One power, one strength, one force within me. I am that I am!

Repeat all the above until you feel centred within yourself. This exercise can be done anytime throughout the day. However one of my favourite exercises can also be done after the Solar Radiance cleansing, if you wish, and that is an abbreviated version of the diamonds of light.

DIAMONDS OF LIGHT

This is another strengthening and balancing exercise, and can be done after cleansing, or on its own. If you think of your aura around the outside of your body having a bright golden chakra (like a golden ball of light) at the top of the aura, another golden chakra at the bottom of the aura below the feet, a golden chakra at the left side of the aura, and one at the right side. Then one at the front and one at the back, near your midline. (all about 4-6 inches out from the body.) Join these chakras up like a diamond, connected by golden lines of light, and you inside the diamond of golden light.

DIAMOND OF LIGHT AFFIRMATION

When you have visualized yourself as the diamond of light command:

"**I am** a Diamond of pure Light"

"**I am** a Diamond of pure Strength"

"**I am** a Diamond of pure Harmony"

"**I am** a diamond of pure Balance.

"**I am** a Diamond of pure Spirit"

"**I am** a Diamond of pure Love"

"**I am** a Diamond of pure Spark of God"

"**I am** that I am"

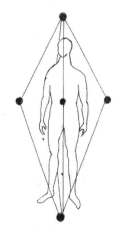

"My true self is now coming forward into the light to achieve all things."

"Beings of Light, Guardian Angels of the Light, please come forward into my life now, to help me in my life, and to help my family, and others. May help also flow out to (name) or others if it is divinely allowable. Thank-you."

Take time to practise these exercises, so eventually your whole being will respond in seconds. These are my favourite exercises, and they have helped me throughout my life even when I sometimes felt I had no hope. I was able to keep strong, keep persevering, keep following my dreams, as I am still doing, with the help and the information from The Beings of Light.

Remember that the Beings of Light, and the Angels of Light love you, want the best for you, and your family, and for all of us. If we can utilize this knowledge, use the herbs, and make a difference, we can truly become empowered. We can feel happier and stronger, and this will radiate out to uplift others.

The Beings of Light have also advised that if we wish, we can also visualize the Solar Radiance flooding into our own gardens once a week for cleansing and to replace the levels with harmony and balance. The Fairies, elves, sprites, plant, air and earth devas, butterflies, insects, and plants will love you for it. It will help them feel more alive, vibrant, and happy, especially knowing that you have the desire to look after nature, the earth and the water. Life is truly magical and wondrous to behold.

LOVE OF THE DIVINE ESSENCE

Another absolute favourite exercise for my friends, patients, their families, and myself is the meditation, "The Love of the Divine Essence." Whenever we are feeling out of sorts, out of balance, or need help, we can place a request to the Beings of the Divine Essence to come in and help us. Think of brilliant white light enveloping you like a waterfall of light as you request:

1. "May the Love and Light of the Divine Essence flow and increase within me." (repeat a few times to feel the energy)

2. "May the Love and Light of the Divine Essence flow, and increase into the area around me." (repeat 1-3 times). (You'll feel wonderful)

The Beings of the Divine Essence will flood you with energy and bring you into harmony and balance quickly. This is helpful if you have to counsel someone, listen to, or talk to, someone who is upset, depressed, tired, or angry. The energy also softens your words, and allows them to flow easily. You may also say after the above:

3. "May the Love of the Divine Essence flow with every word that I speak,"

   or:

4. "May the Love of the Divine Essence flow out to this person to send help into their life, if it is divinely allowable. Thank-you." (or for help in your life)

Remember that we are requesting to the Beings of the Divine Essence, and so they know what help is allowed, or needed, and what Angels may be sent in to help. That's why we must say—" if it is divinely allowable". I have seen wonderful things happen for my children, friends, and patients. I love it, that we can ask for help for others, and The Beings of the Divine Essence love it too.

COMFORTER BEING TO THE LIGHT BLUE

When my children were sick or upset from something which happened at school, when my father had cancer, or my mother had had an operation, I was impressed to bring in the light blue Comforter Being to comfort and soothe them whilst they were sleeping. I request for myself also, when needed. (when I am exhausted, when I broke a bone, or for my cats. The energies are very gentle, and we are allowed to request of this beautiful healing Being:

"Comforter Being to the light blue, please envelop this child with your light blue energies so they may feel comforted, soothed, and nurtured, Thankyou."

You may repeat this request a couple of times as you think of a bubble of pale light blue enveloping your child, or yourself (or pets). This is very helpful in times of stress, feeling drained, sick, anxious, or can't sleep. It is very nurturing.

ARCHANGEL OF LOVE

Although there are many meditations I use regularly, this meditation is soothing, when you need something extra special. In times of severe anxiety, worry, nervousness, loneliness, fear, or stress, or if feeling quite alone, please use this exercise, which was given to me once when I really needed it. This meditation always gives me a feeling of a huge, beautiful Angel enveloping me with his soft, strong wings, and nurturing me with his amazing spiritual love and concern. It has helped me through the toughest times when I had felt that all hope was lost, or when I needed to keep going, or if I felt that even family were not there at the time. This meditation has helped me to feel loved, supported, and cared for, so please use it yourself. Request:

"May an Archangel of Love from the Hierarchy of the Archangels of Love levels, please flood my whole being with your spiritual love and nurturing energies, so I may experience them and feel comforted. Thank-you."

Sometimes I repeat the request, whilst lying in bed at night, and the energies flow quite quickly, so that it is impossible not to relax and be soothed to sleep. Most times the Angels do not seem either male or female, just strong, beautiful, and caring, radiant beings, so to say he, or she, may not be correct.

PROTECTOR BEING

I have included this exercise, as I have found it very helpful on many occasions to ask for protection. One time I was told that we all have many Angels of protection with us, however to just call this one the Protector Being. I have asked the Protector Being to stand outside my house, when I was scared, (especially in a new house) and to also stand beside my bed whilst I am sleeping. Rarely do I feel scared driving, but I was once, whilst being followed at night on a country road. When I asked the Protector Being to come in and help, the other car suddenly sped off. Many times when my son hadn't come home from a nightclub and I had a funny feeling, I asked the Protector Being to make sure he was okay. About ten minutes later he arrived home by taxi and he said he had felt the Protector Being and so came home. When someone was abusive on the phone whilst talking to my child, I asked the Protector Being to stand between them, and the abuser. My child was able to stay calm and speak without intimidation, and told me they felt happy that they could speak up easily. When scared, or whenever you need help quickly, just ask:

"Protector Being please stand beside me (or in front of me) to protect me from harm."
"Thank-you."

Remember to still take all the usual precautions such as locks, and so on.

EXPLANATION OF WORDS AND LEVELS:

1. Dross—this is a buildup of energies, any energies which make us feel drained, or like being enveloped in a heavy cloud. They can be energies of the planets and constellations, heavy positive ions in the atmosphere, too many thoughts and emotions building up in the air, or the radiation from lights and noise at the shops and more.

2. Negative energies—anything which makes us feel tired and not ourselves.

3. Thought forms—a buildup of thoughts in the mental levels, in the atmosphere, or within us. It may be bombardment from the media, or constant chatter from shopping centres, public transport, or just our own mind constantly racing, overthinking, and not being calm. This creates a heaviness, which affects our thinking and our physical body.

4. Emotional forms—similar to thought forms, but a buildup of the emotions in the Astral/ Emotional levels (in the atmosphere or within us), from the media, from our own emotions etc. which causes tiredness, a heaviness, and inability to think properly.

5. Commands—a silent thought, giving direction to an energy or colour, telling it what to do. Commands must be positive, and for the good, for ourselves and our families. They must not be negative, bossy or controlling or they will invert and come straight back to you and cause problems.

6. Cleansing—is needed because we can become out of harmony and balance daily, by being drained and depleted. We can drop down into the lower chakras, not have much energy, not think clearly, not feel positive due to dross, thought forms, emotional forms, and negative energies enveloping us. Also because of:

    a. Bombardment of some planetary or constellation energies, or changes in these energies throughout the day.

    b. If we are sick, tired, anxious, stressed, worried, fearful, or overworked.

    c. Situations we have to deal with in everyday life, such as family or work situations. It may be family patterns, (ie. to be a worrier) or karmic life patterns.

    d. Or we just want to feel better.

BEINGS OF LIGHT

The Beings of Light are coming forward to help us now in our everyday lives. They exist in all levels, all dimensions, and all worlds, and associate with all colours. When using these energies, it is important to use the "light colours," as they are working on a life force level here, and are gentle and uplifting. The dark colours, sometimes relate to strong emotions we have held deep inside us, but aren't ready to face them yet. They can be from a past life, or from childhood, but often, may be unknown. (they can be ascertained by a counsellor or a practitioner who is trained in this area.) Using the "lighter" colour can help by raising the emotions temporarily up into a higher chakra, or by helping to uplift our spirit, awaken the lifeforce, and raise the vibration of our cells.

I have used these colours frequently, when I have needed them, especially when doing talks or seminars for other practitioners, the elderly, students, anxiety groups, and others, as I am usually a very shy person. The Beings and the colours help me to stay calm, and focused, and express easily the words that are needed to explain ideas or guidance. We can help others if they ask for our help or if they are our family. But please always remember never to use any information to affect others against their will, or to manipulate them, as the energies may invert and only adversely affect yourself, and it won't be the Beings of Light that will work with you.

BEINGS OF LIGHT TO THE COLOURS

1. Being of Strength to the Light Red.

2. Being of Harmony & Balance to the Light Orange.

3. Being of Joy and Communication to the Light Yellow.

4. Comforter Being to the Light Blue.

5. Being of stability and calmness to the Light Green.

6. Being of creativity to the Light Violet

7. Nurturer Being to the Light Pink.

There are many more colours and levels, but this is a wonderful and exciting beginning.

1. BEING OF STRENGHTH TO THE LIGHT RED.

The high spiritual Being of Light to the light red can come in to help us when there is a lot to do, and we are feeling tired. We may be fearful of facing up to a situation, and want to have determination, energy, perseverance, and to stop procrastinating. We can then place a respectful request:

"Being of Strength to the Light Red light, please allow your light red light, instilled with the energies of vitality and strength, to flow within every part of my being, and all of my cells so I may have the vitality and strength to study for my exams."

> or a. to clean up the house/ shed/ office/ garden today.
>
>   b. to know how to speak up at this meeting with competence & balance.
>
>   c. to know which direction or pathway to take.
>
>   d. to speak up to my family. (use the Light Yellow after the red.)
>
>   e. to have more energy and determination. (to get a job done)
>
>   f. to feel more competent and alert.

Allow the energies to flow within you until you feel more vitalised, then place a sincere thankyou, and ask that the colour ceases its flow, and any excess is flowing out of you. (just to make sure it doesn't build up too much)

2. BEING OF HARMONY & BALANCE TO THE LIGHT ORANGE.

The light orange light lifts us out of the lower chakras into a higher state of mind, to feel balanced, harmonized, and happier. When desired, request:

"Being of Harmony and Balance to the Light Orange Light please allow your light Orange Light to flow within every part of my being and all of my cells, to build harmony, balance, and happiness within them." (1-5 min.)

When you can feel the change place a respectful thank-you and ask that the colour ceases its flow. You may also request the light orange for:

> a. Balance and clarity.
>
> b. self esteem and balance
>
> c. for balance and healing.
>
> d. to feel happiness and calmness. (to remove any dull feeling.)

Practise this exercise and note any other changes in your body. Your cells will work together better, and be more in harmony with each other. Enjoy!

3. BEING OF JOY & COMMUNICATION TO THE LIGHT YELLOW.

With the light yellow light you should feel lighter and happier, and be able to speak calmly and easily without nervousness or worrying about which words to use. (as some of us are visual, tactile, etc. we use different words and this may cause people to get the wrong understanding of what we are saying.) I always think the yellow makes me feel like whistling, singing, dancing, or having a skip to my step. Yellow is helpful, not only for speaking, counseling, and studying, but also for writing essays, poetry, painting, or any creative expression. (With poetry or music, you could use the light violet Being before the yellow Being.)

You may think of a column of light yellow light coming down from the sky, enveloping you, then request:

"Being of Joy and Commmunication, please allow your light yellow light to flow within my whole being and all of my cells, so I may have better communication and speaking skills". (1-3 mins.)

You may request for:

    a. "happiness and upliftment."

    b. "feeling the joy to be alive."

    c. "joy and vitality."

    d. "creativity and imagination." (for an essay etc.)

Then when you feel the difference, place a sincere thank-you and ask that the colour cease its flow.

This is especially good for counsellors, speakers, therapists, communicators, to have a better balance of words to express your knowledge or guidance. Also for when:

    a. Feeling "low" or like a "cloud" is enveloping you—to let the "light" in.

    b. Helping us feel we did get out of the right side of the bed.

    c. We want to feel an enjoyment of life (or towards others) (it's a happier, balanced way, ie. not false)

d. Feeling too stuck, or grounded, or boxed in.

e. Feeling drained and tired. (also make sure you exercise and eat properly.)

Practise with this beautiful Being of Light, and colour, and note how you feel and how your body and cells respond, so when you need that energy you know when to ask for help. You could say it is like letting the sun in—into all your cells. Have fun!

4. BEING OF STABILITY & CALMNESS TO THE LIGHT GREEN

When too much is going on, or if we are feeling too anxious, too impatient, too nervous, or the mind is overactive, or if we can't sleep, then the light, medium green, and the associated Being of Light, can help tremendously to calm the nerve endings, and relax the muscles and the body. Also when we have too many decisions or choices to make, need centreing, or need to be cool, calm, and collected. For any situation, where we need to stay calm, balanced, and stable, place a respectful request:

"Being of Stability and Calmness, please flow the light medium green light within my whole being and all of my cells, to bring stability and calmness within me." (1-5 mins. or longer.)

When you feel cool, calm and collected, place a sincere thank-you, and ask that the energy ceases its flow. The request can also be used for:

a. "soothing, calming, and relaxing, all my cells." (good for insomnia.)

b. "soothing and calming, all my anxiety, and nervousness." (especially good for fear of planes, heights, roller coasters etc)

c. "soothing and calming my impatience, and irritability."

Once, when I took my teenagers to a Movie fun-park and they told me to go on a little train ride—which it was at first—but it then dropped away into the biggest roller coaster. As I have a fear of these rides I thought my heart was going to jump out of my skin, and that I'd have a panic attack. Luckily, with the help of this Being and the light medium green, (I asked continuously, so I could stay calm) I got through it. Mind you, I love planes, and have no trouble there. Of course my teenagers thought it was hilarious, and said "See Mum, you were OK."—I didn't let on. Of course with teenagers, the green is quite helpful when communicating with them (to stay calm) followed with the light yellow. Try it yourself!

5. COMFORTER BEING TO THE LIGHT BLUE

The comforter Being to the light blue light is a very gentle calming, soothing, balancing, and relaxing energy. It does not give the grounding and stability like the green, as it is lighter in vibration and works on a more subtle level.

As previously mentioned, I love this energy to help me sleep, because it calms the mind, stopping it from thinking all night. It also calms anxiety and relaxes the physical body. By calming the body's nerves and cells it allows healing to take place on many levels. The light blue can be helpful for calming moods, anger, irritability and impatience. Sometimes we don't even know why we feel irritable. (puberty, PMT, menopause anyone?) Although diet, B vitamins, magnesium and chamomile can be calming, you can also ask the Comforter Being and the light blue calm the emotions and nerves. Place a request:

"Comforter Being to the Light Blue Light please flow the light blue within my whole being and all of my cells, to calm, soothe, and balance, my mind and emotions."

Think of a column of blue light enveloping you for a few minutes, then, when you feel the change, place a sincere thank-you, and cease its flow. (if you haven't already fallen asleep.)

I have found the light blue to be very helpful with my birds, and animals and with hurt wildlife. They love it. Then the way they look up at me, I sometimes wonder if they see the Comforter Being with them.

6. BEING OF CREATIVITY TO THE LIGHT VIOLET

The Being of Creativity to the light violet light can be used to awaken our spiritual creative energies, and our latent creative energies within. It is also helpful for writing, poetry, and music, especially on a more ethereal level, so a lightness and wistfulness may be felt. When this energy is needed, place a sincere request:

"Being of Creativity please flow your light violet light into my whole being and all of my cells, for creativity and enlightenment to flow within me, so I am able to be creative and express my ideas more easily." (1-3 mins.)

When you feel the change, place a sincere thank-you, and request that the colour ceases to flow.

    a. You may keep this colour within you longer, for ideas to flow, but then request to cease it and bring in the Being of Light with the light yellow for expression on the material level.

b. This energy helps you to rise above any heaviness and to flow up into our knowing/creative mind. It will also start to awaken your higher mind so it can begin working in harmony with your normal mind.

c. The Being of Light to the light Red can be used after the light violet to give you perseverance, and determination to awaken your spiritual abilities, and to encourage you to practise meditation exercises without giving up.

d. The light violet can be used also with the Being of Light to the light medium green, to have calmness and substance, (or a slight grounding) with your creativeness or expression.

As this colour is quite enlightening, be careful before you drive a car, so always command "I am now returning to my normal self." Or use the green afterwards, so you are grounded.

These colours are only a guideline, practise with them and the Beings of Light. If you ever want to know which Beings of Light and colours would suit you best as an individual, then an experienced practitioner skilled in this knowledge should be consulted. Always listen to your inner mind and inner heart and the Beings of Light who work with you, as to what you think is right for you. You mustn't give your inner power away to others. Enjoy the light and love from the Beings of the Divine Light, who want to help us.

7. NURTURER BEING TO THE LIGHT PINK

The Being of Light to the light pink light, brings in nurturing, soothing feelings of gentle self-love, self-worth, and kindness towards ourselves. These soothing feelings will radiate out from all of our cells into our aura, and then radiate out from our being, and others will feel better too.

Often we may have, locked inside our memory, past events, unwanted feelings or emotions. Perhaps it was when someone had been unkind, demeaning, or was ridiculing us. It may have been from a past life or from this life, as a baby or as a child. The words we heard may have been misinterpreted. In our present life, this can create a feeling of low self-esteem, feeling unappreciated, or even thinking that we are unable to draw, do mathematics, travel, or follow our dreams. All of our cells, as well as our whole being, need this nurturing and soothing pink light from the Beings of Light. It helps us to feel capable and worthy, to overcome the challenges, and achieve our goals, in this lifetime.

We love the idea of cuddling, soothing, and nurturing our children, pets and loved ones, but do not think of nurturing ourselves. We need to feel that spiritual love and nurturing. Place a request:

"Nurturer Being to the Light Pink light please flow the light pink light within my whole being and all of my cells so that I may feel nurtured, loved and comforted."

Think of light pink flowing into your whole being, until you feel a change. (1-5 mins.) Then place a thank-you, and ask that the colour cease its flow.

This meditation brings in a gentle appreciation of oneself, and a feeling as if every cell in your body has a bit of a glow. The light pink is especially good for nurturing the heart cells and immune cells, and other areas that need healing. (remember to still have your herb teas and supplements as they are nourishment on a physical level.)

When feeling stuck, and unable to follow your dreams, try the light pink first, to feel deserving of your dreams, and then the light yellow to communication, to express your dreams and start planning them.

The pink light also helps us to also feel harmonious with other life forces such as animals, birds, plants, the environment, and other living things.

(However, if threatened, by a ferocious animal, immediately bring your Protector Being in, and the Being of Communication to the light Yellow, so the light yellow will flow on the words you speak.)

Although there are many Beings of Light, they are all delighted to come into our lives to support us, nurture us and protect us. Many times in my life they have helped when help was needed most. Enjoy their colours, their divine light and their divine energies.

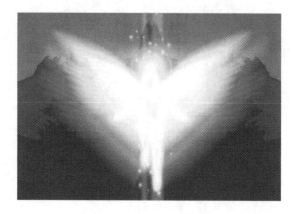

For more information go to:
www.jenniferbailey.com.au

- Which herb, angel and fairy are specially associated to you?

- For personal medical intuitive readings. May also include which herbs, homoeopathics and supplements your body may need.

- Find out who your personal guardian angel is.

- Who is your protector angel?

- Which colours are your own personal health colours, for optimal wellbeing, balance and alignment?

- Animal health and animal medical intuitive readings. May include information about the physical body, their thoughts, and emotions.

- Specific colours, energies and meditations for cleansing your home and garden as well as the ground meridians.

- Meditation lessons to awaken your spiritual energies and knowledge.

- Past life readings. Learn how past lives may affect your health, your emotions, habits, anxieties,

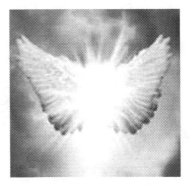